MW01515025

Diabetes

Tragedy

to

Triumph

LESSONS FROM 40 YEARS OF BEATING THE ODDS

DIABETES TRAGEDY TO TRIUMPH

DIABETES TRAGEDY TO TRIUMPH

LESSONS FROM 40 YEARS OF BEATING THE ODDS

by
Tracy Herbert

Diabetes Tragedy to Triumph

Copyright © 2016 by Tracy Lee Herbert

ISBN: 978-1-943767-59-5

eISBN: 978-1-943767-60-1

All rights reserved. No part of this book may be reproduced or transmitted in any form or by any means without written permission from the author.

Printed in USA

Dedication

To my mom for getting up early every morning to pack my lunch (even counting out my olives) and putting up with me not wanting to get up early to check my urine. You must have been scared with my diagnosis, but you never let me see your concern. Dad and Janeece, thank you for continuing to take me out for dinner after my diagnosis, and even though we didn't know what we were doing, you put up a brave face and gave me courage. To my wonderful husband Fred, I am blessed and honored to be your wife. To Josh and Sammie, words cannot express my love and admiration for you—I am one blessed mom! Toni, Miki, and Rachel, having you as daughters is such a joy, and I love you all.

To everyone who reads this book, don't lose hope! Take control of your life today.

Forward

Living with Type 1 diabetes is never easy, and as someone who grew up and witnessed the struggles and lifestyles that came with it, my views of not only diabetes but also how each family member and loved one can be affected was changed as well. My mother has shown that living with this disease for almost 40 years is not a death sentence or an excuse to give up on life and everything you want to do. Instead, it is a new lease on life that, at any age, can be the life you want. She has grown wiser each year and has learned not only a more holistic way to approach this but a lifestyle change that can be easily adapted. She is a hero, a fighter, and a mentor for those of any age affected by this disease.

Josh Bennett (son)

I shouldn't be here. If my mom had listened to what the doctors told her so many years ago and gave up with her diagnosis, I **would not** be here.

I have witnessed my mom take charge of her own health and live the fullest life that she could have envisioned for herself and her family. She has achieved so much through her determination that having diabetes does not define who she is. She is so much more than that; she is, by far, the best mom EVER.

She instilled in her family her passion for healthy living, an active lifestyle, and living every day to the fullest. I am humbled by how much she continues to grow as a person and a mentor. I hope that her intelligence, life experience, and positive outlook give you the determination and a starting point to become your best self as well. If anyone can inspire you along your journey, it's my mom, my hero.

Thanks, Mom, for everything. I love you.

Sammie Bennett (daughter)

Table of Contents

Introduction

"Almost a third of all Americans with pre-diabetes or diabetes don't know they have it. Get the facts on this serious disease, as well as tools for prevention and management."
Dr Mehmet Oz

It is impossible to miss the news reports, advertisements, and people talking about the epidemic rise in diabetes in this country and around the world. It should not come as any surprise when you consider the rise in obesity and our love of video games, television shows, fast food restaurants on every corner, and temptations at every checkout stand from grocery stores to convenience stores, along with sitting long hours at the office every day that diabetes is rampant. When I was diagnosed with Type 1 diabetes in 1978 (called juvenile diabetes then), few people even knew what diabetes was. This book is to help educate in layman's terms and encourage the reader to make changes now before it is too late. The strategies outlined in this book will help you to either prevent, reverse, or control your diabetes.

Diabetes is a collection of diseases characterized by a high blood glucose level resulting either from impaired insulin production or improper insulin functioning or both. Insulin is the hormone produced by the pancreas in the human body and is necessary to mobilize and utilize the glucose derived

1

from food. An elevated blood sugar level, also known as hyperglycemia, is the major effect of diabetes, which, progressively over time, damages many areas of the body, especially blood vessels and nerves.

Diabetes is a global problem that poses serious health consequences for those affected by it, and the disease burden is growing rapidly worldwide. Diabetes is a multi-system, chronic disease that affects millions of people all over the world, and it carries a high death rate while producing various complications. According to the latest (2014) report of the World Health Organization (WHO), it is estimated that about 347 million people are suffering from diabetes worldwide. This emerging epidemic of diabetes can be linked to the increasing trend of obesity and physical inactivity among more and more of the world population. In 2012, 1.5 million deaths worldwide were attributed directly to diabetes. Around 80% of the deaths caused by diabetes occur in middle- and low-income countries. Diabetes is found to be more prevalent among older age groups in developed countries, while in developing countries, it is people between the ages of 35 and 64 that suffer more from it. Fifty to 80 percent of deaths in diabetic populations are due to the cardiovascular diseases that develop as a complication of diabetes. Diabetes has been proven to be the leading cause of kidney failure, blindness, and amputation of limbs all over the world. Currently, diabetes is the eighth leading cause of death in the world, and according to WHO, diabetes has been predicted to become the seventh leading cause of death globally by 2030.

Rise Of Diabetes In The US
Data from tthe Center For Disease Control

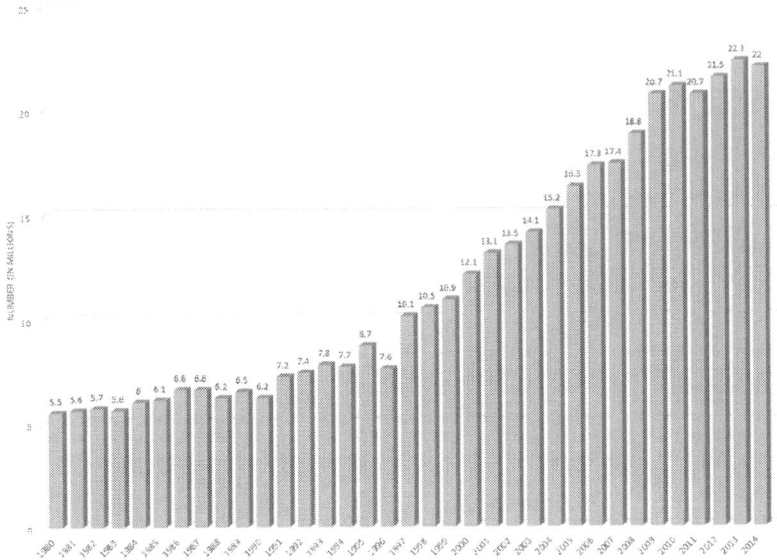

The chart above from the Center of Disease Control clearly indicates the rapid rise of diabetes over the past three decades.

This chart from CDC data shows the percentage of people in each state that currently have diabetes.

State	%
Alabama	11.8%
Alaska	7.6%
Arizona	9.1%
Arkansas	11.5%
California	9.9%
Colorado	6.9%
Connecticut	8.0%
Delaware	9.7%

Florida	9.4%
Georgia	11.0%
Guam	11.6%
Hawaii	8.9%
Idaho	7.0%
Illinois	9.4%
Indiana	9.7%
Iowa	8.3%
Kansas	9.5%
Kentucky	11.3%
Louisiana	10.4%
Maine	7.8%
Maryland	9.2%
Massachusetts	8.8%
Michigan	9.0%
Minnesota	7.5%
Mississippi	11.9%
Missouri	10.0%
Montana	7.6%
Nebraska	8.4%
Nevada	8.8%
New Hampshire	7.8%
New Jersey	8.6%
New Mexico	10.4%
New York	9.2%
North Carolina	9.8%
North Dakota	8.0%
Ohio	10.3%
Oklahoma	10.9%
Oregon	8.0%

Pennsylvania	9.6%
Rhode Island	8.3%
South Carolina	10.7%
South Dakota	8.2%
Tennessee	11.7%
Texas	10.8%
Utah	7.7%
Vermont	6.9%
Virginia	9.0%
Washington	8.2%
West Virginia	12.0%
Wisconsin	8.0%
Wyoming	7.8%

About 29.1 million Americans are estimated to have diabetes, according to the National Diabetics Statistics Report published in 2014, which was based on health data collected from 2012. This constitutes 9.3 percent of the total U.S. population of 318.9 million. The report further shows that out of the 29.1 million estimated diabetics, 20 million were diagnosed with diabetes and 8.1 million were undiagnosed. It has been projected that 208,000 people younger than 20 years old are diagnosed with diabetes. The number of people with pre-diabetes is found to be quite alarming. About 86 million Americans age 20 or older are found to have pre-diabetes. Without taking necessary steps like weight loss, exercise, and dietary modifications, 15% to 30% of pre-diabetics develop Type 2 diabetes within five years. In the USA, diabetes is the seventh leading cause of death, and it has been estimated that

over 1.4 million Americans are diagnosed with diabetes each year.

Diabetes consists of the following types:

o Type 1 diabetes
o Type 2 diabetes
o Gestational diabetes (developing during pregnancy)

Type 1 and 2 are the main types, with Type 2 being the most common and most prevalent. Type 1 typically occurs during childhood or adolescence, whereas Type 2 usually occurs in people aged 45 years or older. However, Type 2 diabetes is now increasingly being diagnosed in children and adolescents and can be related to trends like heredity, obesity, and physical inactivity. Necessary steps should be taken both at the individual level as well as on a global scale to prevent the risk of a rapidly increasing epidemic of diabetes among the masses.

Chapter 1
My Personal Tragedy to Triumph Story

"Do you have diabetes or prediabetes? The choice is yours, you can be a statistic or a success."
Tracy Herbert

I was sick for several months, losing weight, tired, extremely thirsty, and therefore constantly going to the bathroom. After visiting the family doctor, I was told to "drink less ice tea" (even though it was not sweetened, he thought drinking ice tea caused my extreme thirst). I went to the doctor on several other occasions, completed many tests, and was told nothing was wrong with me; the doctor implied it was all in my head. One day while watching TV with my best friend, we started watching Phil Donahue (a popular TV talk show host in the 1970s), and they were discussing juvenile diabetes (now called Type 1 diabetes). We looked at each other and said, "That's it." I was so happy to have figured out what was wrong with me but didn't really listen to the rest show to find out what the disease really entailed. We called the family doctor the next day, and the nurse did not think it was possible (even though I had all the classic symptoms) since no one in my family had diabetes but scheduled me the next day anyway for a blood test. The following day we got the phone call to go to the hospital immediately. We stopped along the way so I could have a hot fudge sundae (my favorite treat), not realizing the grave situation I was actually in. Upon arrival at the hospital, I was swiftly taken to ICU, where I stayed for several days until I could be considered stable and moved downstairs to a standard room.

Almost 40 years ago the technology for dealing with diabetes was in its infancy. The doctors, nurses, psychiatrist, and psychologist were not at all encouraging. They told me I would be lucky to live another 20 years, would not be able to have children, and would die of horrible complications. Being a high school senior, all of a sudden my goals, dreams, and plans were quickly shattered.

It all began with practicing giving shots to an orange before giving them to myself. I was also emotionally overwhelmed with the realities and fears of the complications that I was told would eventually kill me. During my hospital stay, I had extensive training in the current knowledge of nutrition and soon found myself learning the importance of exchanging one type of food for another (this was long before carb-counting became the acceptable practice for people with diabetes). Leaving the hospital, I had no hope.

During my stay in the hospital, I was required to attend multiple support groups. The group consisted of two older men (probably in their 40s and considered "borderline" diabetic) along with myself, who was 17 and had just been given a life sentence of multiple shots daily, not being able to have children (remember the movie *Steel Magnolias?*), and all the other horrible predictions along with the death sentence they had provided for me. One man in my group was complaining about having to cut back on certain foods, while I was practicing the art of giving myself shots and realizing I was not able to eat the normal teenage diet. Being scared, immature, and shaken, I had enough of his complaining, stood up, and said, "I would give my right arm to have your problems and not have to give myself shots for the rest of my life and eat 1,200 calories of food a day, to be able to have children, and to live as long as you have." I stormed back to my room fuming.

I constantly asked myself, *Why me? Why is my life over?* Fear and panic gripped every waking thought. That evening the man who had been complaining in our support group stopped by my hospital room and apologized while thanking me for "opening up his eyes." It was at that moment I found my true passion of helping, encouraging, and, when necessary, being bold enough to help prevent, reverse, and control their diabetes. During the entire 11-day stay in the hospital, I never received any hope or even a single encouraging word. I left the hospital full of fear and hopelessness!

The first six months was difficult. I dealt with depression and high and low blood sugars (this was before the invention of home blood glucose testing), all while being a teenager and trying to fit in. For my first outing with friends after my diagnosis, we went to a movie. I so wanted to be normal and went up to the concessions counter to ask for a cup for a glass of water (this was before diet drinks were available with the exception of Tab, which was only available in cans for home consumption). They told me they could not just give me a cup; even though I offered to pay full price, they still said no. I left the movie theater in tears and decided my life was never going to be good again. I also remember a time going to a friend's birthday party and everyone feeling sorry for me because I couldn't have any cake. Just one of many parties that I left in tears.

Being the hard-headed person I am, depression moved in to resolve that "this isn't going to kill me, and the complications will not win." I started going to the library and tried to keep up with the latest research and up-to-date information. Back then you tested your ketones with a litmus test of your urine. Then the transition was made from urine testing to a finger prick, selecting a color as close to the vial as possible to see the correct indicator of my blood sugar level. With this process, it was almost impossible to maintain good blood sugar control. It was at this point I started giving back to the community by visiting kids in the hospital and offering help to those recently diagnosed. Nurses and hospitals would call and ask me to come speak with the children recently diagnosed and their parents. I was determined to encourage and offer hope to everyone diagnosed with diabetes. It was important to me to provide positive encouragement, unlike the experience I received from the hospital and doctor's office.

While pregnant in 1983, I received my first home blood glucose machine. It was the size of our family Bible, and I was thrilled at being able to see what my readings actually were instead of having to guess. By this time, I was taking three and four shots a day with horrible control. Even with this improved technology, during my first pregnancy, I was rushed to the emergency room 17 times with dangerously low blood sugar readings. One minute I would be having a discussion, and the next minute I would not know who I was because my blood sugar level had dropped so low I couldn't even tell you my name. With my second pregnancy, I had learned how to better control my blood sugars. By the time I hit my mid-thirties, I was getting even more tired and out of control but did not have any of the complications I had been told to expect. I still ate pretty healthy, exercised continuously, and was a mom to two healthy, active elementary school-aged children, but I started to think maybe the experts were right and my time was running out.

In my early 40s, things started to change rapidly. I met and married the love of my life, I was learning about the importance of low glycemic eating, I started exercising the smart way, and I went on an insulin pump. This was another huge breakthrough in my almost 30 years of living with diabetes. I started finding freedom that I didn't think possible. One of my first vacations with the pump was backpacking to the bottom of the Grand Canyon, spending four nights under the beautiful stars, and hiking out on the sixth day. It was so much easier having my pump from a control point of view.

Almost 30 years after my diagnosis, I received the next modern medical miracle, a continuous glucose monitor. Not only did it give me more freedom but, it allowed me more peace of mind while doing life. The alarms alert me to either going high, falling too quickly, or going above or below the safe zone as well as reading my blood glucose every five minutes.

After many hours of research, I realized that even though the medical community considered my diet extremely healthy, I wasn't eating the right way. At this point, I started learning and understanding how food really affects blood sugar.

My desire to make a career out of helping others live a healthy lifestyle all began when I met "Mary." Being 40 pounds overweight with no self-confidence, afraid to go to a fitness center, a hardworking single mom, and "sick and tired of being sick and tired" caused her to have no hope. I offered to meet her at the local track and walk with her. After several weeks of walking and encouraging her, I noticed big changes in her mindset and fitness level. After giving her advice from my experiences with healthy eating and activity, I realized the importance of helping others learn to live healthy. I soon became a certified personal trainer and trained wellness coach and went back to school to get a bachelor's degree in psychology. Realizing the importance of psychology and healthy living, I wanted to go deeper in understanding how the mind impacts our ability to live a healthy life. Now my time is spent working with clients in all walks of life to help them learn the simple strategies to healthy living.

Things I have accomplished since I should have died according to the doctors and nurses:

- Watched both of my children (which I wasn't even supposed to be able to have) graduate from college
- Competed in a triathlon
- Competed in countless 5Ks, 10Ks, and bicycle races/rides
- Became a grandmother
- Wrote a book
- Traveled internationally
- Took numerous backpacking trips
- Graduated college
- Took a weeklong white water rafting trip in the Grand Canyon
- Spoke numerous times about living with diabetes (TV appearances, radio, American Diabetes Association, conferences)
- Encouraged numerous people on how to live successfully with diabetes

"I was determined to share my positive approach and not let diabetes stand in the way of enjoying my life."
Paula Deen

For more resources go to:
www.tracyherbert.com/book-resources

Chapter Notes / Action Items

Chapter 2
What Is Diabetes?

*"When I work, a lot of times I have to lose weight,
and I do that, but in my regular life I was not
eating right, and I was not getting enough exercise.
But by the nature of my diet and that lifestyle -
boom! The end result was high blood sugars that
reach the levels where it becomes Type 2 diabetes.
I share that with a gazillion other people."*
Tom Hanks

Pre-diabetes

Pre-diabetes is a condition in which blood sugar is above normal levels but not high enough to be classified as diabetes. Pre-diabetes can be referred to as borderline or a precursor of diabetes as it can become full-blown diabetes within a decade. Pre-diabetics are the people that are prone to developing Type 2 diabetes mellitus later in their life. According to an estimate, 15% to 30% of pre-diabetics develop Type 2 diabetes within five years. Appropriate lifestyle changes and effective measures can definitely help prevent this progression. However, pre-diabetes is an alarming condition that should never be overlooked as it can develop into serious consequences.

There are no specific signs and symptoms of pre-diabetes. One probable sign that can often be seen in someone with pre-diabetes is the pigmentation of certain areas of the body, causing darkened skin of the respective area, such as elbow, armpits, neck, knees, and knuckles (known as acanthosis nigricans). Pre-diabetes can appear for the first time with signs and symptoms similar to Type 2 diabetes, which indicate that the person has moved from pre-diabetes to diabetes (refer to the Type 2 diabetes section of this chapter).

Similar to diabetes, the diagnosis of pre-diabetes is made on the basis of simple blood tests. Pre-diabetes is also identified as "impaired fasting glucose" and "impaired glucose tolerance." These are identified with the help of blood tests. The following three tests are commonly used for this purpose:

○ **Hemoglobin A1C Test** (also known as average blood sugar test)

This test measures Hemoglobin A1C levels in the blood, which show the average level of blood glucose in the past three to four months. This test can help in the diagnosis of both diabetes and pre-diabetes. However, in diabetics, this test helps in determining the control of blood sugar (whether good control or not). According to the National Institute of Diabetes and Kidney Disease, the test report is interpreted as follows:

➢ Below 5.7% – Normal
➢ 5.7 to 6.4% – Pre-diabetes
➢ 6.5% or above – Diabetes

o **Fasting Plasma Glucose Test (FPG)**

FPG is done in a fasting state (i.e., you are not allowed to eat for eight hours prior to taking a blood sample for the test) and is usually done in the early morning before breakfast. When the test result shows higher fasting glucose levels, the person is exposed to increased risks and complications that are associated with high glucose levels. The test results in context of blood glucose level are interpreted below:

➤ Less than 100mg/dl – Normal
➤ Between 100–125mg/dl – Pre-diabetes or impaired fasting glucose
➤ 126 mg/dl or higher – Diabetes

When the FPG test shows a blood glucose level of 100–125 mg/dl, this refers to impaired fasting glucose, according to the American Diabetes Association (ADA). The WHO values for impaired fasting glucose are somewhat different (i.e., 110–125 mg/dl).

o **Oral Glucose Tolerance Test (OGTT)**

This is another test used for the diagnosis of pre-diabetes. The first part of the test is similar to the fasting plasma glucose test as your fasting blood sugar is measured first on the test day followed by ingestion of 75g of a sugary mixture. Two hours later blood glucose levels are measured again.

If OGTT shows a blood glucose level between 140 and 199mg/dl two hours after taking the sugary mixture, pre-diabetes is diagnosed. This is referred to as "impaired glucose tolerance," or IGT, which is synonymous with pre-diabetes.

A blood glucose level higher than 200mg/dl as measured by OGTT describes a case of diabetes. However, the result can be regarded as normal when blood sugar is less than 140mg/dl after the standard sugar load.

It may be difficult to assign one single cause to pre-diabetes as a variety of factors, including genetics, environmental, and family history, appear to play an essential role in its development. Pre-diabetes develops when the body in unable to properly process glucose anymore and the condition is consistent with impaired insulin usage. Insulin is a hormone produced by the pancreas, which is located in the upper abdomen. Insulin is released upon ingestion of carbohydrate-containing food as it helps to mobilize glucose into the cells, and in this way, insulin helps prevent buildup of glucose in the bloodstream. Pre-diabetes and diabetes are said to result when this normal mechanism of insulin is disrupted at any level, such as insufficient insulin production or inefficient insulin usage by the cells (also known as insulin resistance), producing higher blood glucose levels.

The underlying risk factors leading to pre-diabetes are similar to those causing Type 2 diabetes mellitus. Well-established risk factors that make a person likely to acquire pre-diabetes include the following:

o Age 45 or higher
o Obese and overweight people having a BMI above 25
o Sedentary lifestyle and physical inactivity
o Family history of Type 2 diabetes
o Having an African American, Hispanic/Latino, Asian American, American Indian, or Pacific Islander racial or ethnic background
o History of gestational diabetes during pregnancy or having given birth to a baby weighing 9 pounds or more (macrosomic baby)
o Women having polycystic ovarian syndrome (PCOS), a condition characterized by obesity, hirsutism (excess body hair), and irregular menstrual periods
o Sleep disorders (as they increase insulin resistance)
o Cardiovascular diseases
o Hypertension
o Low HDL (high density lipoprotein), raised triglyceride levels, etc.

The most serious complication of untreated or overlooked pre-diabetes is the development of full-blown Type 2 diabetes mellitus. Other complications that might arise as a consequence of it include hypertension, raised cholesterol levels, stroke, heart disease, kidney disease, blindness, amputations, etc.

The following lifestyle interventions are effective in managing pre-diabetes and preventing pre-diabetes from developing into diabetes:

o **Dietary modifications**
Consume meals that are low in sugars and refined carbohydrates. Limit intake of total calories, sugars, starchy foods, and processed foods, and increase fiber content in your food (see chapter five on smart eating and low glycemic diet).

o **Weight Reduction**
Overweight and obese people are at greater risk for their pre-diabetes turning into diabetes. Research shows that reducing as little as 5% to 10% of body weight has a significant impact on managing pre-diabetes.

o **Physical Activity**
Regular exercise can help prevent and manage pre-diabetes, diabetes, and several other diseases. Get at least 30 minutes per day, five days a week, of physical activity, such as cycling, swimming, brisk walking, etc., to reduce your risk of developing diabetes (see chapter six on smart movement).

Type 2 Diabetes

Type 2 diabetes mellitus, previously known as adult onset diabetes as well as non-insulin dependent diabetes mellitus

(NIDDM), is the most prevalent type. More than 90% of people with diabetes suffer from Type 2 diabetes mellitus, which is a chronic condition characterized by high blood sugar levels produced either due to inability of the cells to utilize insulin or relative lack of insulin in the body. Type 2 diabetes is usually preceded by pre-diabetes, and it has a close association with obesity and metabolic syndrome (a condition comprising of obesity, high blood pressure, and raised cholesterol). The principal factors responsible for Type 2 diabetes include obesity, a sedentary lifestyle with a lack of exercise, and heredity. The typical age of onset for Type 2 diabetes is middle age or older but can also arise in younger age groups. It is thought that Type 2 diabetes reduces up to ten years of a typical life expectancy. (By following these simple strategies outlined in this book, you have the potential to beat these odds like I have.) It is a progressive condition that develops over many years.

Insulin resistance is the primary mechanism causing Type 2 diabetes. Insulin is a hormone produced by beta cells of the pancreas, which acts on the cells of the body and mobilizes glucose into the cells, where glucose is used as a fuel for energy. In Type 2 diabetes, cells of the body become increasingly ineffective in employing insulin to perform its normal functions, and this condition is referred to as insulin resistance, which results in the accumulation of higher levels of glucose in the bloodstream. As cells become resistant to insulin, beta cells of the pancreas try to overcome this by producing larger quantities of insulin; over the span of years, they eventually wear out, leading to insulin deficiency. Thus, in Type 2 diabetes, both the failure of cells to utilize insulin and insulin deficiency co-exist. Risk factors responsible for the development of Type 2 diabetes are similar to those of pre-diabetes (see the previous section on pre-diabetes).

Signs and symptoms of Type 2 diabetes progress slowly over a period of many years (perhaps as a person moves from the stage of pre-diabetes towards diabetes). The most common signs and symptoms of Type 2 diabetes are listed below:

o Polydipsia (increased thirst)
o Polyphagia (increased/constant hunger)
o Polyuria (frequent urination)
o Fatigue and weakness
o Blurring of vision
o Unexplained weight loss or weight gain
o Impaired or slow healing of wounds
o Recurring infections
o Numbness or tingling of hands and feet

Diabetes is also diagnosed on the basis of blood tests showing random blood sugar levels of 200mg/dl or higher, and/or fasting blood sugar level of 126mg/dl or higher, and/or OGTT showing a value of 200mg/dl or higher as well as Glycated Hemoglobin (HbA1c) test (A1C level of 6.5% or above on two separate occasions shows diabetes). Once diabetes is confirmed, further analysis is conducted to differentiate between Type 1 and 2 as both have varying consequences and management. The most important of such investigations is testing for antibodies that are found to be absent in Type 2 diabetes as it is a non-immune condition.

There are various other tests that can be used to differentiate between Type 2 diabetes and Type 1.

Screening for Type 2 diabetes should also be conducted in selected individuals, particularly in overweight children starting at the age of 10 and repeating every two years in addition to adults that are overweight (having a BMI of 25 or above) with other risk factors. Those over the age of 45 years should have the test repeated every three years.

Type 2 diabetes is a life-long illness that poses several threats to health. It is a disease that affects nearly every system in the body. Developing over many years, several serious complications may arise as a result of Type 2 diabetes:

o Eye problems such as loss of vision or night blindness and even total blindness. Every person with diabetes and over the age of 12 should have an eye examination yearly to look for the changes that could lead to diabetic retinopathy.

o Heart problems such as heart attack, uncontrolled hypertension, and sluggish blood flow to the extremities as well as a potential risk for developing cardiovascular disease and stroke

o Damage to the kidneys (diabetic nephropathy) requiring repeated dialysis or even progressing to kidney failure

o Damage to nerves, causing pain, tingling, numbness, and burning sensations. Peripheral neuropathy may arise in which the nerves outside the nervous system (peripheral nerves) stop working properly due to the damage caused by repeated high blood sugars. Damage to the nerves of the gastrointestinal system may cause diarrhea, a bloated feeling, nausea, vomiting, or constipation.

o Foot problems such as non-healing ulcers and even amputations
o Skin problems such as recurring infections
o Sexual dysfunction

Some doctors believe there is no permanent solution for Type 2 diabetes; however, similar to pre-diabetes, Type 2 diabetes is partially preventable by adopting certain measures, such as proper diet, weight reduction, and regular exercise. Apart from lifestyle modifications, Type 2 diabetes is managed with the help of certain diabetes medications. There are several classes of anti-diabetic drugs available, of which metformin is considered as the preferred drug to be used in Type 2 diabetes. If oral medications along with lifestyle modifications do not help reduce the blood glucose levels, insulin can also be added to the treatment. Weight reduction surgery can also be considered in a select group of obese individuals that are unable to control their weight and diabetes otherwise. (I am typically opposed to weight reduction surgery, but if this is the only option to prevent diabetes, then it should be considered.) Preventing the development of complications in Type II diabetes requires thorough attention.

Type 1 Diabetes

This is the kind of diabetes I was diagnosed with at the age of 17. It is believed by the medical community that a virus attacked my pancreas, causing my diabetes. This book is about turning the tragedy of my diagnosis into triumph by beating the odds, and I encourage you to do the same. There is no cure for Type 1 diabetes, but this entire book is focused on living healthy by practicing smart movement and smart eating along with a smart mindset to beat the odds.

Type 1 diabetes, also known as juvenile diabetes, is more prevalent among children and young adults, and it comprises approximately 5% to 10% of all the patients with diabetes. Type 1 diabetes results from very low or absent insulin production by the pancreatic beta cells, which may be destroyed due to autoimmunity or other reasons. Several factors are thought to play a role in the pathogenesis of Type 1 diabetes, such as heredity, immunity, and exposure to certain viruses, etc. However, this kind of diabetes has no cure and there is no prevention, but it can be managed effectively.

The exact cause of Type 1 diabetes remains unknown; however, there are several theories that can explain its origin. Type 1 diabetes may arise as a result of one or more of the following triggers:

o Autoimmunity – Type 1 diabetes is an autoimmune condition in which the immune system (the body's natural guard against harmful microbes and pathogens) considers the pancreatic beta cells to be harmful by mistake and starts destroying them as a natural protective mechanism, which results in insufficient insulin synthesis. What triggers the immune system to behave in such a way is not exactly known; however, it is considered to be due to some viral infection.

o Genes are also thought to play a role in causing Type 1 diabetes as it runs in families. Several such genes have been identified so far.

o Environmental factors as well as certain chemicals and drugs are also thought to cause juvenile diabetes.

o Pancreatic problems, such as trauma, pancreatitis, and tumors, may also lead to loss of pancreatic tissue and thus deficient insulin production, thereby causing Type 1 diabetes.

Several known risk factors are implicated in causing Type 1 diabetes:

o Positive family history of diabetes, such as people having a sibling or parent with Type 1 diabetes

o Young Age - Type 1 diabetes most commonly arises during two age peaks: between 4 to 7 years of age and among children 10 to 14 years of age.

o Genetics - The presence of certain genes makes a person more susceptible to developing Type 1 diabetes.

o Geographical area -Incidence of Type 1 diabetes mellitus is more common among people living away from the equator, so geography may be considered as one factor leading to Type 1 diabetes.

o Other possible risk factors for Type 1 diabetes may include exposure to certain viruses, such as CMV, EBV, mumps, and Coxsackie virus, low levels of vitamin D, neonatal jaundice, and early exposure to cow milk antigens, improper weaning of children, mother with a history of pre-eclampsia during pregnancy, and drinking water containing nitrates.

Type 1 diabetes often has subtle symptoms, but sometimes emergency signs may appear, such as coma (rare), confusion, rapid respiration, fruity smell in breath, and abdominal pain. People with Type 1 diabetes usually experience the following symptoms:

- o Amplified/extreme hunger
- o Increased thirst
- o Frequent urination: This may appear as bedwetting in children whose nights were usually dry previously.
- o Unexplained weight loss
- o Blurring of vision
- o Prolonged and labored breathing (also known as Kussmaul breathing)
- o Weakness and fatigue
- o Increased susceptibility to infections

Type 1 diabetics also are at increased risk for developing a serious condition known as diabetic ketoacidosis that may even lead to coma. Diabetic ketoacidosis (DKA) arises as the body is unable to use glucose as fuel and breaks down fats instead, liberating chemicals called ketones. The accumulation of ketones in addition to glucose building up in the body and dehydration gives rise to DKA, which is potentially life threatening if not treated immediately.

Similar to Type 2, Type 1 diabetes can cause damage to major organs, including blood vessels, nerves, eyes, heart, and kidneys. However, keeping the blood glucose within the normal range can prevent or delay life-threatening complications.

Type 1 diabetes has no cure, but it can be managed by regular administration of insulin and lifestyle interventions which include exercise, proper diet, and regular monitoring of blood glucose levels.

Using appropriate measures and insulin therapy, people with Type 1 diabetes can manage to live a longer, healthier life. The basic goal of managing Type 1 diabetes is to keep the blood sugar levels within the normal range by taking multiple daily injections of insulin or delivery via insulin pump. Depending on the onset and duration of insulin, various types are available:

o Rapid-acting insulin
o Regular- or short-acting insulin
o Intermediate-acting insulin
o Long-acting insulin

Combinations of different insulin injections are used to maintain normal blood glucose levels. People with diabetes should be managed by an expert diabetes care team, and a regular follow up is always required. Modern technology continues to change, including alternatives to insulin injections:

o Insulin pump therapy

o   Transplantation of pancreatic islet cells

o   Transplantation of whole pancreas

People suffering with diabetes require careful monitoring of health and blood glucose levels as it helps to prevent future complications and contributes to a healthy life. Adopting the following measures assists in combating diabetes effectively:

o   Health education: Understand diabetes.

o   Realize it can happen to you.

o   Be compliant with the medication.

o   Maintain regular monitoring of blood glucose.

o   Continue regular follow up with the diabetes medical team.

o   Consume healthy foods and adopt healthy eating practices – Eat foods that are rich in fiber, proteins, healthy fats, fruits, and vegetables while avoiding processed foods, extra salt, unhealthy fats, starchy and high glycemic foods, and sugar.

o   Exercise regularly.

o   Avoid smoking and limit alcohol intake.

o   Take appropriate vaccinations.

o   Take good care of feet and wounds.

o   Have eye examinations yearly or as prescribed by your doctor.

o   Seek help and support.

o   Don't lose hope.

"There are people who could watch a hurricane like Sandy blow out of the Atlantic every other day and blame it on anything but human activity. They are like those who, having been diagnosed with diabetes, eat donuts for breakfast. There's not much to do about them."
Michael Specter

For more resources go to:
www.tracyherbert.com/book-resources

Chapter Notes / Action Items

Chapter 3
The 3M Formula to Beat Diabetes

"My diabetes is such a central part of my life... it did teach me discipline... it also taught me about moderation... I've trained myself to be super-vigilant... because I feel better when I am in control."
Sonia Sotomayor

The following three chapters cover **The 3M Formula.**

- o **Mindset**
- o **Mouth**
- o **Move**

In the image below, mindset is the largest cog because it is the first and most critical step for change. Once the mind adapts, then eating and exercise will quickly follow. Together the three pieces are synergistic and critical in preventing, reversing, or controlling diabetes.

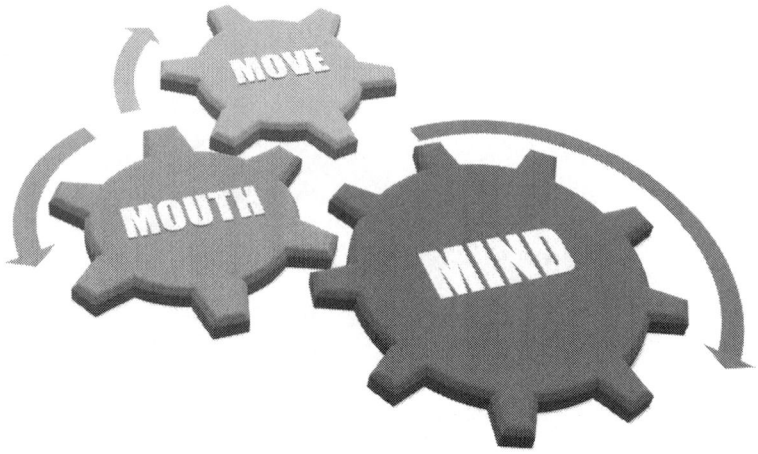

All three work closely together, and if you continue to eat junk food and continue to live a sedentary life, it will affect your mind and sabotage your ability to make the progress you desire.

Mind-Body Connection

It has long been recognized that there is a strong connection between the mind and the body. If one is neglected, the other will suffer. Your body responds negatively to emotions and eventually doesn't work properly when something isn't right. The problem with this is that we try to bury our heads in the sand while hiding our emotions from ourselves and others. When a person is dealing with stress, it can lower their immune system response. The connection between stress and other illnesses suggests that stress can weaken the body's immune system. Stress can raise blood pressure temporarily; however, some studies show that stress can lead to long-term high blood pressure. Personally, stress has always been a challenge for me. Several tools I have learned to help beat the negative effects of stress include exercising, reducing or possibly eliminate caffeine, deep breathing exercises, avoiding process foods, and prayer. Since it is impossible to completely eliminate stress, practicing the techniques I've discovered has reduced the impact of stress in my life and health.

Below are just a few health issues that can arise when the emotional and physical state are not in balance:

o   High blood pressure

o   Chest pain/shortness of breath

o   Headaches

o   Loss of appetite

o   Being tired all the time

o   Back pain or all-over aches and pain

o   Constipation or diarrhea

o   Insomnia or sleeping too much

o   Heart irregularities

o   Weight gain or loss

Poor choices that we make on a daily basis could eventually cause the immune system to be weakened, increasing risks of developing serious diseases. This book is about finding the proper balance of Mind, Mouth, and Movement to help **you** have optimum health no matter what your current diagnosis.

I have already shared how my personal mindset has helped me beat the odds. Read the next three chapters to get an in-depth look at the 3M Formula that worked for me along with valuable tools and strategies that you can implement in your daily life. These strategies work! By accepting your current circumstances, along with changing your mindset, you can add years to your life and find happiness that you only dreamed possible.

> *"Life isn't about finding yourself. Life is about creating yourself."*
> George Bernard Shaw

For more resources go to:
www.tracyherbert.com/book-resources

Chapter Notes / Action Items

Chapter 4
MIND - Smart Mindset

*"To ensure good health: eat lightly, breathe deeply,
live moderately, cultivate cheerfulness, and
maintain an interest in life."*
William Londen

Everyone has a different why—what's your why? In my opinion, the mind is the most important of the 3M Formula. When I first found out I had diabetes, my "why" was this disease was not going to kill me, and I was not going to suffer from the horrible complications that I was told were sure to happen.

What is your reason to get healthy? Is it fear, wanting to see your grandkids grow up, traveling after retirement, avoiding complications (this was my number one reason for changing my mindset), watching your children grow up, graduating from college and getting married, or living a healthy, happy, fulfilled life? Whatever your reason, change your belief system now because this moment in time will never happen again. Thinking *It can't happen to me* or *I will take care of it tomorrow* will only cause disaster. Putting your head in the sand or procrastinating could prevent you from changing your life right now and beginning the health journey you deserve.

Below are some of the strategies and techniques I learned and implemented over the years while living with diabetes:

Motivation

Find the true motive why you want to get healthy. Dig deep, and really find the actual reason. Once you determine your true motivation, visualize the "new" you. Can you see yourself living as a healthier person—the new real you? If your goal is to lose weight, imagine yourself at the ideal weight. If you want to start exercising, visualize yourself after six months of yoga, competing in a race, or playing in a tennis tournament you've always dreamed about. Maybe your motivation is to eat healthy so you can increase your stamina. Picture yourself shopping on the perimeter of the grocery store (the healthiest section of the store). Visual imagery works wonders while it allows for "seeing" yourself in the future exactly the way you want to be. Put pictures around your house or office for visual reminders of what you want to look like. What works for me is having the mental image of the 86-year-old couple I met at the bottom of the Grand Canyon. They hike to the bottom twice a year and were a picture of health. That has been my motivating factor.

The Real Reason

Discovering the real reason why you want to make the change is critical. Is it because you truly want to make the change (internal motivation), or is another factor causing you to want the change (external motivational)? When understanding your true motivation for getting healthy, it allows you to understand the fact that you have a better chance of reaching your goals. If you want your blood glucose levels to remain steady because your doctor or family is pressuring you to make the change (external), you are less likely to make the change or stick with it. However, if the reason you want to make the change is because you want to enjoy life to the fullest (internal), then you are more likely to keep the goal and modify your life.

Reward System

Don't think of rewarding yourself with something to eat but instead find things you enjoy that are placed on hold because of busy schedules, and allow yourself the time to indulge in the activity when you reach a goal. For example, you want to start moving more. After two times of going to the gym, walking around the block, and lifting old milk jugs filled with water (great way to save money on weights) for x number of days, treat yourself to 15 minutes of your favorite book or a magazine. Stop thinking of food as a reward, and look for alternatives. For example, enjoy a bubble bath, take a power nap, treat yourself to a massage, pick a movie you want to see, plan a night out with friends, or put a smiley face or star by the goal you have written down and accomplished.

Support

Positive support is critical when changing from an unhealthy life to one of health and power. Find a friend or a family member that will help you with accountability and will be a reinforcement when feeling tempted to fall back into old, bad habits. We all need help once in a while but especially during hard times. Having a strong group of people supporting you will help you to live longer and cope with life challenges, and you won't have to go through life alone. According to WebMD, a recent study suggests that of 1,500 older people who participated in the study, those with a large group of friends lived longer than those without friends by a whopping 20%. When you have a strong, positive, healthy social support, you will have fewer heart problems and immune issues as well as lower levels of cortisol. Having friends also increases the sense of belonging along with providing a purpose in one's life.

Goal Setting

Set one SMART goal at a time, and decide to do it without exception:

o **Specific** - Indicate exactly what will be done. For example, I will spend 15 minutes today meditating and 20 minutes walking outside.

o **Measurable** - The goal should be measurable. For example, I will lose one pound this week by replacing my five soft drinks with water and lemon, and instead of a doughnut each morning, I will switch to an apple (see more on goal setting later in this chapter).

o **Attainable** - Goals must be achievable but difficult enough to stretch beyond your comfort zone. Set yourself up for victory. You can attain almost any goal. For example, I will lose one pound per week for the next five weeks.

o **Realistic** - Make sure the goal is achievable. You must be willing and capable to work towards making the necessary change. You are the only person who can decide how difficult or easy the goal should or will be. For example, I will take the stairs each morning and afternoon to and from my office instead of the elevator.

- o **Timed** – Set a time when you will complete it. Without a timeframe aligned with the goal, there is no sense of urgency. For example, before Sunday I will walk 15 minutes on two separate occasions.

When you reach the first SMART goal, pat yourself on the back, and then start with the next goal. Writing goals down and placing them strategically throughout the house, office, and car will help keep you focused on what is important and help remove any distractions. Using a smartphone reminder will also keep you engaged in the behavior associated with the goals being met. Getting your day started on the right foot will help you to stay positive, goal oriented, and driven throughout the entire day.

Goal-Setting Tips

- o Start with long-term goals (longer than three months). For example, in five months, I will walk in my first 5K (3.1 miles) event for diabetes.

- o The next step is short-term goals (less than three months). For example, in two months, I will walk one mile without stopping.

o Finally, decide on your weekly goals. For example, I will start by walking to the end of the street on Monday, Wednesday, and Friday this week.

o Establish a clear path to reach your short-term goals while on the journey to accomplishing your long-term goals.

o You can reach almost any goal you set when you determine to do it, plan your steps accordingly, and establish a realistic timeframe that allows you to accomplish those steps.

o Monitor progress towards the goals.

o Make sure the goal indicates meaningful and measurable progress.

o Involve family members, your medical team, and friends in helping you reach your goals (pay careful attention to only having those who support and encourage you through this journey).

o Reward progress.

o The biggest problem my clients face with goal setting is failing to set specific goals.

o It might seem at first to take too long to set goals, but it is well worth it. It actually saves time because when setting goals, you become more organized and efficient with time.

o Set just one or two goals since setting too many goals at once will make you feel overwhelmed; this will prevent you from giving up.

o Determine why you want to make the change.

o Prepare in advance to determine what blockades or possible obstacles could arise to keep you from reaching the goal.

o Remember, if you feel overwhelmed, take a deep breath and think about why you are working towards this goal. Don't let negative feelings burden you to believe you can't achieve it

If you don't come up with your "why," you will more than likely stay on the couch and not exercise, you will continue to eat the wrong kinds of food, and you will not make the necessary changes to live a healthy life. Since your "why" is such a motivating factor for success, if you do not know your "why," then make that your first goal.

We've all heard "we are what we eat," but I believe "we think like we eat" too. When we fill our bodies with processed foods and not vegetables and fruit, it affects our minds. Several studies have found a correlation between a diet high in processed foods, fast foods, high fructose corn syrup, and sugars and weakened brain function along with the development of depression.

Someone with Type 2 diabetes is much more likely to develop depression than those without diabetes. According to the Center for Disease Control, having diabetes doubles your risk of becoming depressed. So the question being addressed at this time is, are people with diabetes more susceptible to depression because of the illness itself (high blood sugar levels) or because of dealing with the chronic disease on a daily basis. If you think you might be suffering from depression, seek help immediately. Don't go through this battle alone. People who have diabetes and are depressed typically have higher hemoglobin A1c levels and a higher rate of suicide. Another scary fact is that those with depression and diabetes have larger healthcare costs compared to those without depression. People with blood sugar levels that are not in control often show some of the same classic symptoms as someone who is depressed. The medical community needs to be diligent when trying to determine if it's depression or diabetes.

Coaching

There is value in getting the help of an expert who can coach and encourage you through the transformation. Professional athletes, along with other successful people, hire coaches to help them reach their goals. A good coach will listen to you, encourage you, challenge you, motivate you, help you make better decisions, and guide you to the healthier life you desire.

I have been coaching for many years and have seen remarkable changes in my clients. If you find yourself recently diagnosed, stuck, and not getting the results you desire, a health coach might be exactly what you need to get you over the hump.

Finding the right coach can be a challenge. Be sure to talk with several coaches before deciding on one. This may sound self-serving (since I am a diabetes coach), but I feel that having a coach that truly understands is extremely valuable. Having dealt with diabetes (Type 1, the most challenging) for almost 40 years successfully without complications, this puts me in an ideal position to guide anyone with prediabetes or Type 2 diabetes. Consider me if you need help and get to the point where you need a coach to help you reach your health goals: http://tracyherbert.com/

While it starts with Mindset, they work so closely together that if you don't eat or move properly, it will affect your mindset and sabotage your ability to make the progress you desire.

Mind Body Connection
It has long been recognized that there is a strong connection between the mind and the body. Your body responds to your emotions and tries to tell you when something isn't right. The problem is we often try to block our emotions from ourselves and others. It is very common to hear of someone dealing with high blood pressure or an ulcer when going through a

very stressful time in their life. For example, I went for several years in a very high stress job and actually caused my heart to skip a beat. It is better now that I am removes from the stressful environment but this is a clear case of my health being affected by my mental state.

The list below is just a few of the known health issues that can be caused when your emotional and mental state are not in balance:

o   High blood pressure

o   Upset stomach

o   Back pain

o   Loss of appetite

o   Chest pain

o   Constipation

o   Diarrhea

o   Extreme tiredness

o   General aches and pains

o   Headaches

o   Sexual problems

o   Insomnia

o   Lightheadedness

o   Heart palpitations

o Shortness of breath

o Stiff neck

o Sweating

o Weight gain or loss

Your immune system can be weakened by your poor emotional health and increase your risk of developing a serious illness.

This book is all about finding the proper balance of Mind, Mouth, and Movement to help you have optimum health no matter what your current diagnosis.

I have already shared how my personal mindset has helped me beat the odds. I am living proof that it can be done and I urge you to take these next chapters very seriously and do whatever you can to find the balance that will add years to your life and life to your years.

The future you see is the future you get.
Robert G. Allen

For more resources go to:
www.tracyherbert.com/book-resources

Chapter Notes / Action Items

Chapter 5
MOUTH - Smart Eating

One should eat to live, not live to eat"
Benjamin Franklin

Smart eating is critical to having good health. When I was first diagnosed in the 1970s, I was taught the importance of the exchange diet (exchanging one food option for another) and was not allowed to eat anything with sugar. As a teenager, I thought my life was over. At that point in my life, I hadn't learned the importance of "eat to live, not live to eat." Fast forward 25 years and I had resigned to a life of multiple shots a day (up to seven), and if I wasn't eating lunch by 11:25, my blood sugar level would drop so low that I wouldn't even know my name.

The solution for my abnormal low blood sugar would be to drink a tall glass of orange juice. This would start the beginning of the roller coaster. The orange juice would quickly raise my blood glucose level, which would improve my cognition, but then for the next four or five hours, my blood sugar levels would be so high I would need to take another correction (aka another shot). This went on for several years until I decided enough is enough. After researching numerous books and articles on eating healthy and what causes blood glucose levels to rise, I quickly realized why I was so tired mid-morning after eating a bowl of cereal with milk. What I didn't realize at the time is how much my blood glucose levels were rising each morning with the heavy carb breakfast I consumed and therefore creating unnecessary blood sugar spikes and causing me to feel tired and lethargic while beginning the ups and downs of living with diabetes.

It was at this point that I discovered the importance of eating a low glycemic diet. By practicing a low glycemic eating plan, my blood glucose levels began to become steady, with the additional benefit of losing weight. A typical eating plan that I follow for most meals is 65 percent low glycemic vegetables, 15 percent protein, 10 percent low glycemic fruit, and 10 percent healthy fats.

Low Glycemic Diet
It has been known for many years that diabetes can be best managed by following simple measures such as good diet, regular exercise, and a healthy weight. Among countless diets, a low glycemic diet is the best option for people with diabetes, which not only helps keep blood sugar levels in the normal range but also helps in burning fat. A low glycemic diet contains foods that when consumed, cause minimum variation of blood sugar levels. A low glycemic diet is based on the principle of the glycemic index, which determines the amount of blood glucose raised after consumption of a carbohydrate-containing food. Glucose is given the glycemic index (GI) of 100 and is used as a reference food as other carb-containing foods are valued against the GI of glucose. Non-carbohydrate containing foods such as meat and fats have no glycemic index.

GLYCEMIC INDEX

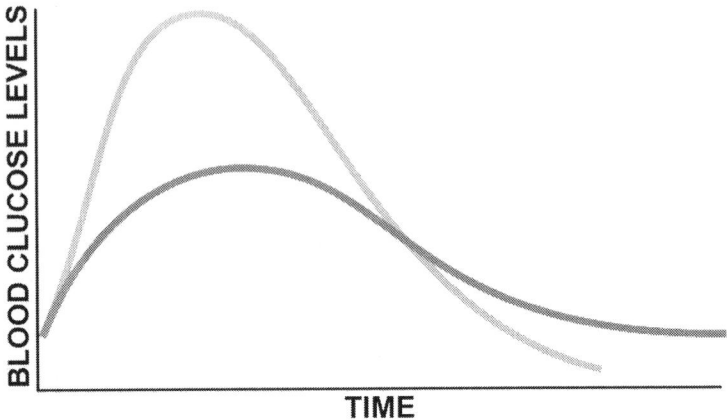

High GI means rapid and more glucose (or energy), while foods having a medium or less GI causes a slower and minor rise in blood glucose. Various carbohydrate-containing foods can be grouped on the basis of GI as follows:

- Low GI = 55 or less
- Medium GI = 56-69
- High GI = 70 or more

While 55 or less is classified as low, my personal belief is that you should try to keep your GI at 40 or below to avoid blood sugar spikes. A low glycemic index diet offers better management of diabetes, enhanced control of blood cholesterol, and therefore a decreased risk of heart (cardiovascular) complications. Some foods having low GI include many fruits, nuts, dried beans and legumes (such as kidney beans and lentils), yam, carrots, and all non-starchy vegetables. Some of these starchy vegetables should be eating in moderation like sweet potatoes and many whole grain breads and cereals (such as whole wheat bread, rye bread, barley, and all-bran cereals). Consumption of foods having a low glycemic index results in a steady rise of blood glucose (preventing side effects of hyperglycemia and hypoglycemia), takes longer to digest (helps in controlling appetite), and supports weight loss.

Food with a high GI (70 or more) causes a rapid rise of blood glucose and more release of insulin, which results in fatigue, increased appetite, and poor diabetes control. High GI foods deliver greater amounts of glucose, providing plenty of readily available extra energy in your blood, which is then stored as fat. Foods having a high glycemic index include certain fruits such as melons and pineapple, white bread, bagels, corn flakes, bran flakes, puffed rice, instant oatmeal, white rice, pasta made from rice, macaroni, white potatoes, pumpkins, pretzels, rice cakes, etc.

There are certain limitations to the Glycemic Index as it can only be applied to a single food entity, while food combinations can alter the GI. Sometimes the accurate GI of certain foods is difficult to assign, and basic principles of a balanced diet should also be incorporated while following low GI diets. High GI food should be combined with a low GI food to balance the effect of both on blood sugar level. GI values describe the type of carbohydrate but is of no value in predicting the amount of carbohydrates to be consumed. Total calorie intake along with the size of meal is also important in maintaining a healthy weight and diet.

High GI	70 or greater
Medium GI	56-69
Low GI	<55

Food	GI	HML	Serving Size	GL
CANDY/SWEETS/SNACKS				
Honey	87	High	1 Tbs	3
Pretzels	83	High	30g (1 oz)	16
Jelly Beans	78	High	1 oz	22
Vanilla Wafers	77	High	25g	14
Graham Crackers	74	High	25g	14
Snickers Bar	68	Medium	60g (1/2 bar)	23
Table Sugar	68	Medium	2 Tsp	7
Corn Chips	63	Medium	50g	17
Popcorn, plain microwave	55	Low	20g	6
Potato Chips	54	Low	114g (4 oz)	11
Strawberry Jam	51	Low	2 Tbs	10
Peanut M&Ms	33	Low	30 g (1 oz)	6
Dove Dark Chocolate Bar	23	Low	37g (1 oz)	4
BAKED GOODS & CEREALS				
Corn Bread	110	High	60g (1 piece)	31
French Bread	95	High	64g (1 slice)	30
Corn Flakes	92	High	28g (1 cup)	21
Corn Chex	83	High	30g (1 cup)	21
Rice Krispies	82	High	33g (1.25 cup)	23
Corn pops	80	High	31g (1 cup)	22
Donut (lrg. glazed)	76	High	75g (1 donut)	24
Waffle (homemade)	76	High	75g (1 waffle)	19
Grape Nuts	75	High	58g (1/2 cup)	32
Bran Flakes	74	High	29g (3/4 cup)	13

Food	GI	HML	Serving Size	GL
Graham Cracker	74	High	14g (2 sqrs)	8
Cheerios	74	High	30g (1 cup)	13
Kaiser Roll	73	High	57g (1 roll)	21
Bagel	72	High	89g (1/4 in.)	33
Corn Tortilla	70	High	24g (1 tortilla)	8
Melba Toast	70	High	12g (4 rounds)	6
Wheat Bread	70	High	28g (1 slice)	8
White Bread	70	High	25g (1 slice)	8
Kellogg's Special K	69	Medium	31g (1 cup)	15
Taco Shell	68	Medium	13g (1 med)	5
Angel food cake	67	Medium	28g (1 slice)	11
Croissant, Butter	67	Medium	57g (1 med)	18
Muselix	66	Medium	55g (2/3 cup)	24
Oatmeal, Instant	65	Medium	234g (1 cup)	14
Rye bread, 100% whole	65	Medium	32g (1 slice)	9
Rye Krisp Crackers	65	Medium	25 (1 wafer)	11
Raisin Bran	61	Medium	61g (1 cup)	24
Bran Muffin	60	Medium	113g (1 med)	30
Blueberry Muffin	59	Medium	113g (1 med)	30
Oatmeal	58	Medium	117g (1/2 cup)	6
Whole wheat pita	57	Medium	64g (1 pita)	17
Oatmeal Cookie	55	Medium	18g (1 large)	6
Popcorn	55	Medium	8g (1 cup)	3
Pound cake, Sara Lee	54	Low	30g (1 piece)	8
Vanilla Cake and Vanilla Frosting	42	Low	64g (1 slice)	16
Pumpernickel bread	41	Low	26g (1slice)	5
Chocolate cake w/chocolate frosting	38	Low	64g (1 slice)	12

Food	GI	HML	Serving Size	GL
BEVERAGES				
Gatorade Powder	78	High	16g (.75 scoop)	12
Cranberry Juice Cocktail	68	Medium	253g (1 cup)	24
Coca Cola	63	Medium	370g (12oz can)	16
Orange Juice	57	Medium	249g (1 cup)	14
Carrot juice (freshly made)	43	Low	250g (1 cup)	10
Hot Chocolate Mix	51	Low	28g (1 packet)	12
Grapefruit Juice, sweetened	48	Low	250g (1 cup)	13
Pineapple Juice	46	Low	250g (1 cup)	15
Soy Milk	44	Low	245g (1 cup)	4
Apple Juice	41	Low	248g (1 cup)	12
Tomato Juice	38	Low	243g (1 cup)	3
LEGUMES				
Baked Beans	48	Low	253g (1 cup)	18
Pinto Beans	39	Low	171g (1 cup)	12
Lima Beans	31	Low	241g (1 cup)	7
Chickpeas, Boiled	31	Low	240g (1 cup)	13
Lentils	29	Low	198g (1 cup)	7
Kidney Beans	27	Low	256g (1 cup)	7
Soy Beans	20	Low	172g (1 cup)	1
Peanuts	13	Low	146g (1 cup)	2
VEGETABLES				
Potato, white	104	High	213g (1 med)	36
Parsnip	97	High	78g (1/2 cup)	12
Carrot, raw	92	High	15g (1 large)	1
Beets, canned	64	Medium	246g (1/2 cup)	10
Corn, yellow	55	Medium	166g (1 cup)	62
Sweet Potato	54	Low	133g (1 cup)	12
Yam	51	Low	136g (1 cup)	17
Peas, Frozen	48	Low	72g (1/2 cup)	3

Food	GI	HML	Serving Size	GL
Tomato	38	Low	123g (1 med)	2
Broccoli, cooked	0	Low	78g (1/2 cup)	0
Cabbage, cooked	0	Low	75g (1/2 cup)	0
Celery, raw	0	Low	62g (1 stalk)	0
Cauliflower	0	Low	100g (1 cup)	0
Green Beans	0	Low	135g (1 cup)	0
Mushrooms	0	Low	70g (1 cup)	0
Spinach	0	Low	30g (1 cup)	0
FRUIT				
Watermelon	72	High	152g (1 cup)	7
Pineapple, raw	66	Medium	155g (1 cup)	12
Cantaloupe	65	Medium	177g (1 cup)	8
Apricot, canned in light syrup	64	Medium	253g (1 cup)	24
Raisins	64	Medium	43g (small box)	21
Papaya	60	Medium	140g (1 cup)	7
Peaches, canned, heavy syrup	58	Medium	262g (1 cup)	28
Kiwi, w/ skin	58	Medium	76g (1 fruit)	5
Fruit Cocktail, drained	55	Low	214g (1 cup)	20
Peaches, canned, light syrup	52	Low	251g (1 cup)	18
Banana	51	Low	118g (1 med)	12
Mango	51	Low	165g (1 cup)	13
Orange	48	Low	140g (1 fruit)	7
Pears, canned in pear juice	44	Low	248g (1 cup)	12
Grapes	43	Low	92g (1 cup)	7
Strawberries	40	Low	152g (1 cup)	4
Apples, w/ skin	39	Low	138g (1 med)	6
Pears	33	Low	166g (1 med)	7
Apricot, dried	32	Low	130g (1 cup)	23

Food	GI	HML	Serving Size	GL
Prunes	29	Low	132g (1 cup)	34
Peach	28	Low	98g (1 med)	2
Grapefruit	25	Low	123g (1/2 fruit)	3
Plum	24	Low	66g (1 fruit)	2
Sweet Cherries, raw	22	Low	117g (1 cup)	4
NUTS				
Cashews	27	Low	50g (¼ cup)	3
Almonds	0	Low	NA	0
Hazelnuts	0	Low	NA	0
Macadamia	0	Low	NA	0
Pecans	0	Low	NA	0
Walnuts	0	Low	NA	0
DAIRY				
Pudding	44	Low	100g (1/2 cup)	8
Milk, Whole	40	Low	244g (1 cup)	4
Milk, Skim	32	Low	244g (1 cup)	4
Ice Cream	38	Low	72g (1/2 cup)	6
Yogurt, Plain	36	Low	245g (1 cup)	6
MEAT/PROTEIN				
Beef/Chicken/Fish /Eggs/Pork, etc.	0	Low	NA	0
MISCELLANEOUS				
Pizza, plain with parmesan and sauce	80	High	100g	22
Hamburger, with bun	61	Medium	¼ oz pattie	14
Macaroni and Cheese , Kraft	64	Medium	166g	30
Hummus	6	Low	30g	0

This chart was pulled from multiple sources. The University of Sydney has done exhaustive research and testing and would be a good source for additional information. Here is their website: http://www.glycemicindex.com/

The Right Choice

Maintaining and losing weight is based on burning more calories than the intake of calories. Not all calories are equal, and the impact of metabolism should also be taken into consideration. This can be best achieved by combining a diet providing less caloric intake with an active lifestyle incorporating regular exercise. Glycemic Index should not be used alone in predicting what to eat, and other nutritional factors (total calories, portion size, amount of fats, fiber, vitamins, etc.) must also be taken into account. A diet should be followed under the supervision of an expert. For diabetics and pre-diabetics, low glycemic diets offer several benefits, including blood sugar management, weight reduction, and help in maintaining an active and healthy lifestyle.

As mentioned earlier, my typical breakfast used to be cereal and milk. After researching, learning, and testing new recipes, I quickly realized the breakfast I was eating not only affected my blood sugar levels but also left me feeling lethargic. Now my breakfast has been completed transformed, and I have more energy throughout the morning than ever before. Every morning for breakfast I have a shake consisting of the following: unsweetened almond milk, cube approximately an inch of ginger root, chia seeds, hemp seeds, flax seeds, organic cocoa powder, organic protein powder, kale, spinach, peppermint oil, cinnamon oil (which has been known to help regulate blood glucose levels for certain people with Type 2 diabetes), and ice. Also, each day I snack on a green apple (remember, an apple a day keeps the doctor away) along with nuts, berries, and fresh vegetables. It has eliminated the sluggish feelings I used to experience before making the switch. It also reduces hunger pains and cravings, improves mental clarity, and achieves almost perfect blood glucose levels, which makes me the happiest.

Make the right choices with simple, healthy choices. For example, instead of choosing a medium white potato (which has a GI of 104) choose a sweet potato (having a GI of 54). Why not make the switch to replace some of your higher glycemic foods to lower glycemic foods? Not only will it help you control your blood sugar but it will probably help you reduce body weight and have more energy.

The countries with the typical Western diet, which consists of processed and refined foods and sugars, proves to have more people with depression than those who eat like the Mediterranean and Japanese typical meal plan, which is higher in vegetables, fruits, fish, and seafood and with only small amounts of lean meats and dairy products.

Ditch the soft drinks for tea! According to a John Hopkins study, drinking one cup of black or green tea can slash your risk of heart disease by 35% and reduce the buildup of plaque commonly associated with cardiovascular disease versus those who don't drink any tea. Another benefit of drinking tea is that it can reduce your risk of certain types of cancer and can lower blood pressure and cholesterol. Not to mention the dangers of high fructose corn syrup in regular soft drinks and the toxic chemicals found in artificial sweeteners.

Having a well-hydrated body is critical to a healthy life. If at first you don't enjoy drinking water, add lemon, limes, or a slice of cucumber to give it an added zest. Drinking water also reduces hunger pains. When you feel hungry, most of the time it is because you are dehydrated. Drinking a glass of water before a meal will help you differentiate between true hunger and dehydration. Another benefit of drinking a glass of water before a meal is that it will likely reduce the number of calories you consume. The body is composed of approximately 60% water. Each day we lose water by evaporation from the skin, urine, and breathing. Water is critical to bodily functions such as circulation, digestion, transporting nutrients, and maintaining body temperature. Muscles require adequate fluids to function properly. In order for the kidneys to function properly, an adequate amount of water is necessary. Water is also crucial to prevent constipation. The current recommendations for water intake is half of your body weight in ounces.

Being Prepared

Preparation is the key to making healthy choices. It takes more time up front, but by having healthy choices available at home, at the office, and in the car, it makes it easier to stay on target. For example, I always have a water bottle with me everywhere I go, and I carry almonds, walnuts, and pecans for a healthy snack option. Always have a snack, and drink plenty of water before going to the grocery store. This will help you avoid impulse shopping. Each week I cut up various fresh vegetables and place them in sandwich bags, which helps speed up packing lunches and extra goodies to put in our salads.

Eating a small salad or something healthy before going to a party will give you the power and a feeling of satisfaction before being tempted by unhealthy options that are usually available at parties. Being successful at a party requires decisions before leaving the house. Simply predetermine what you will or will not eat or drink. Prior to going out for dinner, I will commonly plan to eat a salad and protein or other healthy options even though I know my friends and family will choose unhealthy options. This way, by planning before leaving the house, I have a goal and am prepared.

"You can't exercise your way out of a bad diet."
Mark Hyman

For more resources go to:
www.tracyherbert.com/book-resources

Chapter Notes / Action Items

Chapter 6
MOVE - Smart Movement

"Physical fitness is not only one of the most important keys to a healthy body, it is the basis of dynamic and creative intellectual activity."
John F. Kennedy

In this country, we just don't move enough! Sitting disease is the new smoking and is partially the cause of the epidemic rise in Type 2 diabetes and obesity. Some researchers have found that sitting too much can be compared to the ill effects of smoking. In this chapter, I cover the third M in my 3M Formula to beat diabetes. By following these simple suggestions covered in this chapter, you will find strategies to help move from a sedentary life to an active, healthy lifestyle. Having someone you enjoy doing things with will help keep you motivated. Personally, I like to change things up as to not get bored. Remember to start off slow and let your body adapt. Starting too quickly can lead to injury and burnout. Always check with your doctor before starting or increasing an exercise program. Following the strategies below will help jumpstart your road to getting healthy:

o   To prevent sitting too long, set an alarm for every 50 minutes, and get up, stretch, and walk around.

o   Instead of sending an email, walk to their office to discuss the matter with a co-worker.

o In the office setting, consider having walking meetings.

o Get a stand-up desk.

o Stand while talking on the phone. I like to march in place while talking on the phone.

o Get up and move during TV commercials.

o Instead of meeting friends for lunch, take a walking lunch and stop for a salad.

o Park farther away from the door. (Remember. it's not being lucky to get a front row parking spot; it's unhealthy.)

o Take the stairs instead of using elevators or escalators.

Exercise and Diabetes

Diabetes is a chronic disease that demands changes to your lifestyle in addition to sticking to various drug treatments, where appropriate. It is vital that everyone incorporate regular physical activity in their lifestyle, but it proves to be highly advantageous for diabetics and pre-diabetics. Exercise is an important component of the management of diabetes, particularly Type 2 diabetes. People gain several benefits by simply exercising regularly, such as enhanced control of blood sugar, boosting their fitness level, and less risk of developing long-term complications of diabetes.

Research indicates that exercise and an active lifestyle can prevent or delay the onset of diabetes among pre-diabetics and those susceptible to developing diabetes. Many studies over the years have shown the importance of physical activity and exercise in the prevention and management of diabetes, and it is now well recognized that participating in regular physical activity improves control of blood sugar and overall diabetes, along with other added benefits, such as positively influencing lipid management, blood pressure, metabolism, and cardiovascular events as well as fewer incidences of neuropathies and death. Regular exercise has certain health benefits, such as weight loss, stress reduction, better sleep, more energy, stronger muscles, stronger bones and joints (reducing the risk of falling as we age), and fewer chances of developing chronic diseases. Regular physical activity also helps in lowering blood pressure and cholesterol levels, lowers the risk of cardiovascular diseases and stroke, reinforces a strong heart, improves blood circulation, and hence improves the overall quality of life.

How Exercise Reduces Blood Sugar
Blood glucose levels can be efficiently lowered with the help of exercise. Type 2 diabetes is characterized by very high blood sugar level produced either due to inability of the cells to utilize insulin (known as insulin resistance) or due to relative lack of insulin in the body. Insulin is a hormone synthesized by the pancreas, and it mobilizes glucose from the blood into most of the cells in the body (predominantly muscle and fat tissue cells). Within the liver, insulin helps in the conversion of glucose into glycogen by the process of glycogenesis. These

functions of insulin are essential for the control of blood sugar levels. In diabetes, insulin resistance hinders the normal mechanisms of insulin by limiting the cells' ability to recognize and utilize insulin, thus leading to higher levels of blood sugar. Exercise effectively combats insulin resistance by increasing insulin sensitivity of the cells so that cells are better able to utilize available insulin and uptake glucose from the blood, both during and after the physical activity. Enhanced sensitivity to insulin as imparted by the physical activity causes the body cells to take up and utilize the glucose that is present in larger quantities in the blood of diabetics. This effect of lower insulin resistance or enhanced insulin sensitivity remains up to approximately 24 hours or more after the exercise, and it effectively controls blood sugar levels.

Exercise has a positive effect on lowering blood glucose by reducing the amount of insulin needed. During exercise, muscles contract and are able to take up glucose to fulfill their increasing energy requirement by a mechanism independent of insulin. In other words, exercising muscles are able to take up glucose from the blood whether insulin is present or not, and in this way, exercise helps control the blood sugar level. It has also been suggested that exercise may also lead to less need of the drugs usually required to control blood sugar levels.

Prerequisites for Exercise in Diabetes
Exercise can definitely offer several short- and long-term benefits to those with diabetes or prediabetes; however, these effects may not be observed during the initial phases of

starting a physical activity. It takes some time for the human body to adopt and react to new changes. There are certain prerequisites and precautions that should be kept in mind before embarking on any exercise, especially by diabetics:

Consult Your Healthcare Provider

For the effective management of your diabetes, exercise is a must, but before starting any physical activity, it is wise to seek a doctor's help and guidance. Experienced healthcare providers will give guidance about your heart health, which is relevant if you have developed narrowed arteries (atherosclerosis), cardiovascular problems, or hypertension (high blood pressure). They inform you if you need to reschedule your meals, insulin, prescriptions, and workout. Consideration of certain complications of diabetes such as retinopathy and neuropathy is also important as it has been shown that some exercises may worsen eye disease (retinopathy) with diabetes.

Choose a Reasonable Exercise Plan

Set realistic goals, and gradually increase the quantity and intensity of exercise. Stay motivated, and follow a healthy and practical exercise routine. You can also select easy and enjoyable activities such as dancing, aerobics, cycling, tennis, swimming, walking, yoga, working in the yard, and anything that gets you up and moving. Finding a good personal trainer who can provide proper exercise strategies, techniques, and accountability will help push you to the next level of your health journey.

Monitoring Blood Sugar Level with Exercise

It is critical to measure blood glucose levels before, during, and after the physical activity. This helps in predicting the response of the body to the physical activity and dangerous consequences (such as hypoglycemia) that should be considered. Check blood sugar before exercise. During the exercise, blood sugar should be monitored, especially if your physical activity exceeds 45 minutes in duration. After the physical activity, the effects of exercise on blood glucose may persist for 12-24 hours, and blood glucose should be monitored during this time too. It is also advised to keep a snack with you during exercise to be used if any symptoms of hypoglycemia appear. For example, I respond to exercise differently than others with Type 1. It is critical to determine how your body responds to exercise and not what is considered the "norm." While participating in competitive athletic events, my blood sugar levels increase because of my adrenaline and do not begin to drop until 45 minutes or longer after the event is over. Many people with diabetes are just the opposite. This is why it is important to test and track your own blood sugar levels.

Keep Yourself Hydrated
Drink plenty of water throughout the day. Pay special attention to hydrate yourself before, during, and after the exercise. Avoid working out in extremely hot or cold weather conditions.

Take Good Care of Your Feet
Wear proper shoes, and pay special attention to any injuries inflicted on feet. Take proper care of personal and feet hygiene.

Best Exercises for Diabetes

Choose the type of physical activity that suits you and your lifestyle the most. If you enjoy it, you will do it; if you don't, you won't. Do what you love and what's best for you. Always begin with an easy and limited activity, and gradually increase the duration and intensity of the workout. The most popular exercises that are especially helpful for diabetics are given below:

Aerobic Exercises

Aerobic exercises are on top of the list of best exercises for diabetes. The National Institutes of Health (NIH) has suggested approximately 150 minutes of aerobic exercise each week. Exercise is considered so imperative for people with diabetes that the American Diabetes Association (ADA) has recommended that people with diabetes should exercise at least five days a week. Aerobic exercises increase the insulin sensitivity of the body cells. It helps in strengthening the heart, muscles, and bones; relieves stress; improves blood circulation; and reduces the risk for heart diseases by lowering blood sugar, cholesterol, and blood pressure.

The recommended length for a daily aerobic activity is roughly 30 minutes. You can do this time in one segment, or it can be broken down into 10-minute intervals. Aerobic exercises can be listed as follows:

o   Walking (especially brisk walking)
o   Cycling
o   Jogging/Running
o   Dancing

o Aerobics
o Stair climbing
o Hiking
o Tennis
o Basketball
o Swimming
o Gardening
o Yardwork and housework

Strength/Resistance Training
Strength training is recommended once you have integrated aerobic exercises into your routine. It is recommended to practice strength training at least two days a week in addition to aerobics. Strength or resistance training helps build stronger muscles and bones in addition to enhancing insulin sensitivity and lowering blood glucose. It also helps in preventing osteoporosis and bone fractures. Strength training should be practiced for roughly 20-30 minutes a day and two to three days a week.

Strength training activities include the following:

o Weight lifting or training
o Lifting free weights or using weight machines at a gym
o Home workouts such as pushups, sit-ups, planks, lunges and squats, etc.

Balance Training
Balancing can help combat diabetic neuropathy among diabetics. With the development of the complication of neuropathy, it gets more difficult for the patients with

diabetes to maintain normal gait and balance, which is accompanied by loss of sensations, particularly in the feet. Balancing can help people with diabetes in managing such problems. When adequate balance is achieved, falls and injuries can be possibly eliminated.

Stretching and Flexibility Training
Flexibility training, such as stretching, can help in maintaining more flexible and stronger muscles and joints. Stretching before and after a workout can prevent muscle tears, aches, and soreness. Stretching exercises include basic or static stretches, dynamic stretching, moderate yoga, Pilates, Tai chi, etc.

Interval Training
Interval training is adding short periods of high intensity activity into your regular exercise regimen. Interval training helps in improving stamina, effective control of blood sugar, and improving cardiovascular status. Interval training has been around for a long time having been used mostly by athletes, until the past few years. After much research it has been determined that interval training also improves lung function, reduces blood pressure faster than some aerobic type exercises. According to Dr. Joseph Mercola, recent studies have discovered that older adults who are healthy but unfit were able to improve their blood glucose levels and insulin sensitivity after several weeks of interval training. The study goes on to say that "just one interval training session was able to improve blood sugar regulation in people with Type 2 diabetes for the next 24 hours."

Fifteen to thirty seconds of high intensity bursts of activity incorporated into regular training may help achieve the benefits of interval training. Personally, I find this type of exercise most beneficial with my busy schedule and for helping with my blood sugar control. Warm up for three minutes, and then start to exercise as hard and fast as you can for 15-30 seconds. At this point, you should be out of breath and begin to slow back down but continue to move. When starting out, do only two or three high intensity bursts, or as tolerated, and add additional cycles as you get stronger. Remember, cooling down is important.

Below is an example of what I do on my interval training days (especially those days that when time is limited).

Be sure to check with your doctor before starting an exercise program. With interval training, you only want to do it once or twice a week unless an elite athlete. For beginners, just completing two or three interval series will provide a healthy workout option until building up to the full 15 minutes.

Description	Time
Warm up	Begin - 3 minutes
Go as hard and fast as you can safely	3:00 minutes - 3:30 minutes
Slow down keep moving let heart rate come back down	3:30 minutes - 5:00 minutes
Go as hard and fast as you can safely	5:00 minutes - 5:30 minutes
Slow down keep moving let heart rate come back down	5:30 minutes - 7:00 minutes

Go as hard and fast as you can safely	7:00 minutes – 7:30 minutes
Slow down keep moving let heart rate come back down	7:30 minutes – 9:00 minutes
Go as hard and fast as you can safely	9:00 minutes – 9:30 minutes
Slow down keep moving let heart rate come back down	9:30 minutes – 11:00 minutes
Go as hard and fast as you can safely	11:00 minutes – 11:30 minutes
Slow down keep moving let heart rate come back down	11:30 minutes – 13:00 minutes
Go as hard and fast as you can safely	13:00 minutes – 13:30 minutes
Slow down keep moving let heart rate come back down	13:30 minutes – 15:00 minutes
Go as hard and fast as you can safely	15:00 minutes – 15:30 minutes
Slow down keep moving let heart rate come back down	15:30 minutes – 17:00 minutes
Cool down	17:00 minutes – 20:00 minutes

Longevity

There is a strong link between exercise and health, and regular exercise is associated with living a longer life. Even a moderate level of regular movement will help to lower your risk of death. Being physically active helps reduce the risk of obesity, cardiovascular disease, and diabetes and often reduces stress. Putting an exercise program in place is often difficult however. Some of the excuses that are used for not being able to exercise are lack of time, not convenient, and doesn't enjoy it. "Fitness is a journey, not a destination; you must continue for the rest of your life." Kenneth H. Cooper, MD, MPH

Following these steps below will help you get off on the right track:

o   Find something you enjoy—because if you don't enjoy it, you won't do it.

o   Don't overdo it when exercising. If you start off too strong, you will suffer from burnout or injury. You will be more likely to stay with a fitness plan that involves more consistent workouts of moderate intensity than one that is less frequent but more extreme.

    o   Increase the length of time you work out slowly. Slow and steady wins the race, and developing an exercise plan is no exception.

o   It's not too late to start.

    o   According to the Center for Disease Control, only 20.8% of Americans participate in regular exercise, and that percentage decreases with age.

    o   Consider the consequences of not beginning or increasing your exercise regime.

o   Do you suffer from depression? For many people, an exercise prescription is just as effective as prescription medication (without any of the negative side effects).

o Another benefit is that the mental decline slows down by eating healthy and exercising. Who doesn't want to grow old while staying mentally sharp?

o Weight bearing exercise will help with bone loss. Did you know that after the age of 30, bone growth stops and bone loss begins? (Don't forget about the importance of Vitamin D in the supplement chapter.)

  o Brisk walking, running, lifting free weights, or resistant training on machines

o Exercise helps

  o Improves balance (which is critical as we age), helps with weight control, boosts energy, improves mood, helps with sleeping, may ease arthritis, often improves sex life, builds self-esteem, gives a "runner's high" (which is one of the main reasons I enjoy exercising), reduces stress, and helps to prevent, reverse, or control Type 2 diabetes.

"Those who think they have no time for exercise will sooner or later have to find time for illness.'
Edward Stanley

For more resources go to:
www.tracyherbert.com/book-resources

Chapter Notes / Action Items

Chapter 7
Discipline and Self-Control

"You can achieve anything you want in life if you have the courage to dream it, the intelligence to make a realistic plan, and the will to see that plan through to the end."
Sidney A. Friedman

The question I have been asked the majority of the time while living with diabetes is "How do you live with this chronic, difficult disease for as long as you have without getting overwhelmed and burned out?" Another common question is "How do you take care of yourself day in and day out?" Learning discipline and self-control is a lifelong journey. Think of increasing your self-control like developing strong muscles. The more you choose the right, healthy options, the easier it is for you to choose it the next time.

The first few years after being diagnosed, I struggled with depression. Not only was I required to learn the daily struggles of taking multiple shots and managing my blood glucose levels but I also had to stop eating what my friends were eating. In our society, eating is a social activity, and when I was left out because of not being able to eat the typical teenage diet, it only increased my anxiety and depression. However, it also taught me a great deal about discipline. While my struggles caused depression, anxiety, and loneliness, I can look back now and realize this time in my life helped me form the self-discipline that I needed to deal with this disease and outlive my life expectancy.

One of the strategies I have used to keep from being tempted by unhealthy foods is to imagine nails, tacks, and even poison in the food. This completely eliminates my desire for the foods that would keep me from my health journey. Another strategy that works for me is to think if I eat this, then this or that negative consequence will happen. The biggest fear that has been with me constantly is developing one of the many serious complications that go hand in hand with diabetes (refer to the chapter on complications). So the choice is mine—do I fight every day, or do I make excuses as to why I can't exercise, why I should eat that unhealthy food instead of eating healthy and maintaining steady glucose levels, or why I should stay up late and avoid getting a good night's sleep?

Taking control of your life will help you to be more disciplined. Since I have been practicing self-control for so long, it is like a strong muscle that continues to get stronger each day. For example, when I try to talk myself out of doing some sort of exercise, I now ask my today self what my 80-year-old self would tell me today. Without a doubt, I know my older self wants me to work out today so I can continue to be strong and free of typical elderly issues like falling and not being able to take care of myself. As mentioned in the section regarding Mindset, it is apparent that in order to live successfully with diabetes, one must think like a Drill Sergeant.

According to Roy Baumeister, Ph.D., an expert in self-control and willpower, the following three strategies can be employed to help you develop strong willpower:

o Determine the motivation required to achieve the set goal.

o Observe the actions related to the goal.

o Develop the willpower to accomplish the goal.

Keys that I have learned over the years:

o Not only is self-control important for living a healthy life but it also helps improve other areas of your life as well.

o Having a strong emotional support group of friends and family will help you succeed and reach your goals.

o Keep a journal, not just for food choices but also emotional risks and successes.

o Self-control is a personality trait you are born with, but it can still improve and strengthen with simple strategies practiced daily.

o Focus attention away from the attraction that is trying to destroy you or keep you from reaching your health goals. For example, look at a hot fudge sundae (my biggest temptation) and think about it having sharp pins placed strategically in the sundae, or imagine carrying around a bowling ball around all day because of the weight it could cause you to gain. Out of sight, out of mind often works best, especially at first. However, I think it could prevent the strengthening of willpower. If the temptations are too much to bear, then remove the temptation from the house, car, and office.

o Change your thinking from something negative to something positive. Instead of thinking about going to an exercise class as exhausting and hard work, think of the benefits you will feel afterwards, like better mental clarity, improved self-esteem, and added energy.

   o Listen to an exciting audio book, but only listen to it while exercising. It will help you exercise longer to see what happens next. Those that practice something fun while exercising spend 51% more time at the gym than those that do not.

o Change the people you run around with and the locations of your favorite hangout place.

   o If you have always had candy on your desk at the office, get rid of the candy altogether, or place it in the break room. Better yet, bring fresh fruit, nuts, or other healthy snacks.

o Get your friends together, and instead of having an unhealthy lunch, opt for something healthy and walk around the block first.

o Use if...then statement. If I am tempted later today with a hot fudge sundae, then I will turn it down and take 15 minutes to enjoy a nice, relaxing warm bath (or whatever you enjoy doing). Having a strategy in place before the temptation appears helps to avoid a split-second decision that could alter your self-control and will instead help you make choices drawing on your willpower rather than in the moment.

o Another strategy that has worked well for me over the past 10 years is having water with me everywhere I go. When it comes to hunger, at the first hint, drink a glass of water and wait a few minutes. Typically, the desire to eat goes away.

o If eating a low glycemic meal plan the majority of the time, blood glucose levels remain constant and steady. Temptations and bad choices happen frequently before a meal or several hours after eating a high carbohydrate meal. Blood glucose levels and willpower reduction are often tied together. This is why it is important to eat before heading to the grocery store. If weight loss is a goal, you might be better off eating smaller meals frequently throughout the day rather than skipping meals. Also, check with your doctor if you have been diagnosed with diabetes and especially if you are on medication for diabetes.

o Focus on one goal at a time and making it more possible to achieve. Having five or six goals at once often leaves the person feeling overwhelmed, and they frequently give up.

A key component of self-control with diabetes is maintaining good blood glucose levels. Find whatever strategy works best: rewards, distractions, or avoidance. It is up to the reader to discover what works best. Practice these tools, and see how quickly your self-control will strengthen. Living with diabetes is easier with a strong level of self-control. In our society, we want things right now, and unhealthy things are no exception. Developing the ability to delay gratification will help remove the temptations, and they will flee our thoughts and cravings. For example, if tempted to have a cookie at the mall, remind yourself what your health goals are and then walk around for 30 or 45 minutes. After some time has lapsed, you will be shocked to see the temptation to eat the cookie is gone.

Self-discipline is a key strategy in dealing with diabetes and other chronic diseases. Make it your goal to work each day to develop this mental muscle so that you will find that making the right choices will begin to come more naturally and easily over time.

"Life is not over because you have diabetes. Make the most of what you have, be grateful."

Dale Evans

For more resources go to:

www.tracyherbert.com/book-resources

Chapter Notes / Action Items

Chapter 8
Diabetes Complications

"Time and health are two precious assets that we don't recognize and appreciate until they have been depleted."
Denis Waitley

Whatever you do, do not skip this section!

It is difficult reading about all the bad things that can happen; however, since having made the decision to change your mindset, it all starts with knowing it can happen to you and being willing to face the unpleasant facts. Now for the good news, and yes, there is always good news—you are taking the right steps by reading this book and determining to make the positive and necessary changes.

While writing this book, I went back and forth on whether to write a chapter on complications. The biggest fear I have faced over the past 40 years is the possibility of developing these horrific diabetes-related complications. Another factor was my desire to keep this book positive and not oversell the "fear factor." However, using my fears of complications as negative reinforcement, I continue on a daily basis to make healthy decisions and have had zero complications. Understanding that amputations are often a result of having diabetes, it gives me the necessary motivation to go to the gym or find something else to keep me moving. My drive to avoid these complications has motivated me to eat healthy, to find ways to move smart, and to keep a positive mindset to avoid the following complications.

Kidney Disease

Diabetes is the number one forerunner of kidney disease. When someone has diabetes, the small blood vessels in the kidney can become damaged and no longer filter impurities from the blood efficiently. When this occurs, the result is called nephropathy. Once the damage to the kidneys reaches end-stage renal disease, that person is required to go on dialysis. Someone with diabetes is about 20 times more likely to develop end-stage renal disease than people without diabetes. When a person's blood sugar is higher than normal, it causes the kidneys to filter too much blood.

Heart Disease

Diabetes often causes obstructions in arteries and is a major risk factor for heart attacks. People that have diabetes are twice as likely to have heart attacks compared to those without diabetes. Diabetes that is uncontrolled can cause damage to the body's blood vessels, making them more prone to damage from atherosclerosis (formation of plaque around the interior lining of walls). Those with diabetes often develop atherosclerosis younger and more severely than those without diabetes and are more likely to have a heart attack than people that do not have diabetes. Since diabetes can cause destruction to nerves, heart attack symptoms can be less obvious for those with diabetes than the characteristic warning signs, such as chest pain, for those without diabetes.

Stroke

Stroke is a major risk factor for someone with diabetes. If you have diabetes, you are at a one and a half times greater risk of having a stroke than someone without diabetes. Another reason people with diabetes have strokes more often is the fact that several risk factors for diabetes often coincide with other risk factors. A stroke is a brain attack that happens when a blood clot blocks an artery or a blood vessel breaks, interfering with blood flow to a certain area of the brain and therefore killing brain cells. Hypertension (high blood pressure), also a complication of diabetes, is still the leading cause of stroke. People with diabetes have an even higher probability.

Vision Issues

Since diabetes damages the small blood vessels, the retina is no exception. Diabetes is the leading cause of blindness for adults. Diabetic retinopathy causes between 15,000 and 30,000 new diagnoses annually, making diabetes the leading cause of new blindness each year. Having a yearly eye exam will help the doctor check for swelling of the blood vessels and weakening of the blood vessel walls to avoid rupturing of the vessels.

High Blood Pressure

The majority of people with diabetes have high blood pressure. This increases the risk of heart attack, stroke, heart failure, and kidney disease. It is reported by the American Diabetes Association that two in three people with diabetes suffer from high blood pressure or take prescriptions to lower it. When someone has high blood pressure, the heart needs to work harder than for those whose blood pressure is within the normal range.

Amputation

Diabetes is the second leading cause of amputations. The majority of amputations involve toes, feet, and legs. In addition to nerve damage, foot ulcers can become infected to the point that antibiotics or other wound care specialties fail to work, leaving the patient with amputation as the only chance of survival. An amputation at mid-calf increases the risk of death from other diabetes complications. Peripheral vascular disease involves poor blood circulation to the legs and nerve endings. When circulation begins to slow down, cuts are slow to heal, often causing infections, which can lead to gangrene. Approximately half of those with diabetes have some degree of neuropathy.

Nerve Damage

Diabetes produces nerve damage all over the body. Most often it is found in the legs and feet. Numbness, dizziness, diarrhea, tingling, loss of balance, and muscle weakness are common symptoms of nerve damage.

Impotence

As discussed above, having diabetes causes damage to blood vessels and nerves throughout the body. This damage can cause impotence in men.

Celiac Disease

Celiac disease is more prevalent in people with Type 1 diabetes (5-10%) compared to less than 1% of those without diabetes.

Motivated yet?

Allow these possible diabetes complications to motivate you to take this disease seriously and cause you to take action on the strategies discussed in this book. Motivation is part of your **Mind**, which helps make better choices about what you put in your **Mouth** and how you **Move**. There are no guarantees, but your risks will decrease greatly if you follow my 3M Formula. I credit my living with Type 1 diabetes for almost 40 years without complications to the following: my ability to research and learn new ideas and my willingness to try new healthy strategies along with discipline and determination. God's grace, along with my faith, has allowed me to continue in this health journey and live another day to the fullest.

"Good health is not something we can buy. However, it can be an extremely valuable savings account."
Anne Wilson Schaef

For more resources go to:
www.tracyherbert.com/book-resources

Chapter Notes / Action Items

Chapter 9
A Different Approach to Supplements

"Today, more than 95% of all chronic disease is caused by food choice, toxic food ingredients, nutritional deficiencies and lack of physical exercise."
Mike Adams

My first exposure to supplements was about 12 years ago when my husband suggested I start taking a probiotic to help prevent "leaky gut." Not only did I have continuous constipation, stomach issues, and aches but I was constantly getting sick with every virus and ailment that was going around town. At first I didn't notice any changes until I realized that I was no longer getting sick all the time. Over the years I have researched and discovered what would improve my energy level, overall health, and longevity. The list below is what I typically take either daily or weekly. Supplements can be controversial, and remember to always talk with your doctor before taking any of these items below. Also, keep in mind that supplements react differently for different people.

Vitamin D
Vitamin D is a hormone that effects every part of the body. It is reported that over 50% of the population suffers from low levels of Vitamin D. People with lower vitamin D levels are more prone to Type 1 and Type 2 diabetes. A recent study in India found that giving one unit of Vitamin D, along with exercise, reduces the risk of developing Type 2 diabetes by 8%.

It is important that you get the appropriate level of Vitamin D to maximize your health and prevent disease. A John Hopkins study shows that diabetics with poor glucose control are also linked with low levels of Vitamin D. Of course, the best place to get Vitamin D is sunshine, but remember to only stay in the sun the appropriate amount of time for you based on your skin type. Vitamin D can also be found in eggs, cod liver oil (which is what I use), milk, sardines, canned tuna, and supplements.

Probiotics

Probiotic means "for life." Probiotics contain live bacteria and yeast and can help move food through the stomach. According to Harvard Medical, "a growing body of scientific research suggests that you can treat and even prevent some diseases with foods and supplements containing live bacteria." Probiotics are considered safe and help replenish the body's balance when antibiotics, urinary tract infections, and irritable bowel syndrome disrupt the body's balance. Foods with probiotics include natto (Japanese fermented soybeans), Greek yogurt (make sure to watch the amount of sugar), sauerkraut, miso, and kefir. Pickles could also be a choice depending on how they are processed. Some studies suggest that people who take probiotics had improved mental attitudes versus those who did not take probiotics as well as lower anxiety levels.

Vitamin C

According to several studies, those with higher levels of Vitamin C were less likely to develop Type 2 diabetes. This is another supplement with varying views of its importance by the scientific community. Some of my favorite natural sources for Vitamin C are kale, broccoli, Brussels sprouts, cauliflower, kiwi (medium Glycemic Index and low Glycemic Load), bell peppers, and strawberries. Adding Vitamin C to your diet reduces the risk of eye disease, can protect the immune system, and reduces the risk of cardiovascular disease. Unless you eat a large majority of fruits and vegetables, most studies recommend adding a supplement.

Chromium

Some researchers have found that chromium may improve the effectiveness of insulin and therefore improve blood glucose levels along with HgbA1c. A study in a 1997 *Diabetes Journal* article suggests that chromium has "significant beneficial effect" with lowering blood sugar levels. The best low glycemic choices for chromium are broccoli, garlic, and meat.

Magnesium

Deficiency in magnesium has been known to cause heart disease in patients. This is because magnesium can relax blood vessels, therefore lowering blood pressure. Another way to get magnesium in your body is through the following foods: almonds, avocado, kidney and black beans, spinach (refer to the chapter on smart eating for my shake recipe), quinoa, bananas (although bananas have a higher glycemic index and load), lentils, and oatmeal (but not instant).

Fish Oil – Omega-3

According to WebMD, there are different types of omega-3s: ALA (alpha-linolenic acid), DHA (docosahexaenoic acid), and

EPA (eicosapentaenoic acid). Your body can turn ALA into DHA and EPA but not very well. There are no agreed upon standard dosage recommendations in the medical community for how many omega-3s we need. Recommendations range from 500 to 1,000 milligrams (mg) daily. A can of tuna or a few ounces of salmon provides approximately 500 mg. Consuming appropriate levels of omega-3s has been found to lower blood pressure, triglycerides, and cholesterol (lowers LDL and raises HDL) and can possibly help alleviate depression. Several ways to add omega-3s to your diet include eggs, flaxseed, salmon, fresh tuna, walnuts, kale, and Brussels sprouts.

Multivitamins
If your diet is full of many healthy choices, a multivitamin in not needed. However, according to Joslin Diabetes Center, if processed and fast foods are consumed the majority of the time, then adding a daily vitamin might be beneficial. Aim for a vitamin no more than 100–150 percent of the recommended daily value. Men and post-menopausal women should avoid vitamins with iron.

Cocoa
Cocoa has a large amount of epicatechin, which is anti-inflammatory and helps prevent damage to blood vessels, the leading cause of cardiovascular complications (see the previous chapter on complications). Always look for cocoa that is unsweetened and non-alkalinized to get the maximum benefits. It can prevent the effects of aging too.

Cinnamon

Cinnamon has been around since 2800 BC and has numerous health benefits: It can help reduce blood sugar spikes, reduces the speed of emptying of the stomach, lowers cholesterol (cinnamon can prevent damage to arteries because of its anti-inflammatory fighting properties), helps prevent urinary tract infections, helps with indigestion and bloating, and the anti-inflammatory properties help reduce stiffness caused by arthritis.

Flaxseed

Flaxseed can lower blood sugar and cholesterol. Several studies have been recorded, but the outcomes seem to differ; however, the studies have only been associated with Type 2 diabetes. I add flaxseed to my breakfast shake every morning, but it does not affect my blood sugar levels since I have Type 1 diabetes. I use flaxseed in my diet to increase my omega-3s (for heart health), antioxidants, and fiber.

Do your own research, and be your own advocate! In our diets today, it is impossible to get all the nutrients we need from foods alone. These are the supplements I take, and I will continue to research and find other supplements to help improve the quality of life. Science is changing daily, and new studies are continually finding the benefits of certain supplements.

"If you don't take care of your body, where are you going to live?"
Unknown

For more resources go to:

www.tracyherbert.com/book-resources

Chapter Notes / Action Items

Chapter 10
What's Next

*"The root of all health is in the **brain**. The trunk of it is in emotion. The branches and leaves are the body. The flower of health blooms when all parts work together."*
Kurdish Saying

Change your belief system. Thinking that "it can't happen to me" or "I will take care of it tomorrow" will only lead to disaster. Placing your head in the sand or procrastinating could prevent you from changing your life right now and beginning the health journey you deserve.

Tracy's Tips
Over the years I have helped my clients with frequent short and to-the-point health tips. To see more tips on a regular basis, like my Facebook page at:

https://www.facebook.com/tracyherbertcoaching/.

Below are a few of my favorite tips:

○ Start by getting a good night's sleep. A dark, cool room provides the most restful sleep. "A good laugh and a long sleep are the best cures in the doctor's book." Irish Proverb o   Plan to not hit snooze in the morning, and go to bed 15 minutes earlier than usual.

o   Before getting out of bed, find something to be thankful for, and say it out loud. If you can't think of anything, be thankful that you're alive.

o   Each morning drink a warm cup of water with a few lemon slices in it. (It helps remove toxins and flushes out the kidneys.)

o   Spend 10 or 15 minutes praying, reading something positive, or journaling. For me, I read the Bible each day in addition to prayer. Find that one thing that helps you understand that the world is a bigger place than just you.

o   Remember to begin SMART goal setting: Specific, Measurable, Attainable, Realistic, and Timed.

o   Set goals and keep them.

o   Remember, eat to live and not live to eat.

o   Get a big calendar, and each day you exercise, mark the calendar with a star. After several weeks, you will see stars throughout the month, and this will help you visualize the improvements you have made.

o   Find an exercise you enjoy because if you don't enjoy it, you won't do it.

o Start exercising now, which can release endorphins to help you feel happier, and self-esteem will also increase.

o If you have been trying to do it alone and have been unable to get the results you want, hire a coach.

o Eat every three or four hours to maintain blood sugar levels (if on diabetes medication, always check with your doctor before changing your meal plan).

o Remember that processed foods and junk food increase cravings. Avoid the white, unhealthy options: sugar, flour, and salt.

o When you take care of yourself physically, you will also be taking care of yourself emotionally. Negative emotional behaviors create a lethal cycle. Simple strategies like getting enough rest, eating a healthy diet, practicing mindful breathing, and drinking plenty of water can create a new healthy cycle. When you decide to start moving, your mood and attitude will improve. Remember, you do not need to be perfect. The goal should be to be better tomorrow than you are today. Do not compare yourself to others.

Engaging in positive social gatherings is critical. We are social creatures and thrive when socially connected. Whom you spend time with matters. "Your social networks may matter more than your genetic networks. But if your friends have healthy habits you are more likely to as well. So get healthy friends." Mark Hyman

o Community is one of the strongest predictors of a long, happy life. Make sure you have people around you that are positive and strive for the same types of healthy living you desire. Even though we have negative people in our lives, strive to spend as little time as possible with those types of people. Those with stable, positive, and loving family and friends live longer. Grab a workout partner because you will stay consistent in your health goals of moving more when you have someone with you. Those that exercise by themselves stop sooner than those that work out with a friend.

o Take time to relax and enjoy life. Relaxing helps to reduce the risk of stroke (see the complications chapter), can reduce the risk of depression (see the mindset chapter), helps keep the weight off (cortisol increases appetite and even certain food cravings), and can even protect your heart. My favorite way to relax is prayer and meditation. Take the time now to create a stress management plan to prepare for those stressful days. By doing this, you will have action items set in motion before the stress appears. Take time to love yourself—you're worth it! Take a deep breath, and practice mindful breathing.

o Get a good night's sleep. Practice these simple steps to help get the Zs needed for good health: Do the same thing every day, go to bed at the same time and get up at the same time, take a warm bath before bed, and exercise daily but not too close to bedtime. Nicotine and caffeine are both stimulants and take a while to wear off, and alcohol could effect a good night's sleep by waking you up in the middle of the night. Turn off computers, TVs, and phones an hour or so before bedtime. According to the Joslin Diabetes Center, people with diabetes have more sleep issues than those without diabetes. The higher the blood glucose levels, the worse the sleep is. Mark Mahowald, MD, director of the Minnesota Regional Sleep Disorders Center in Hennepin County believes there is a correlation between lack of sleep and the development of pre-diabetes. Also, those that sleep less are typically heavier.

o Be in tune with your body. Know the difference between true hunger pains and either emotional eating or being dehydrated.

"Body listens to mind; mind listens to body. Awareness is the link. Make no mistake: Every cell knows when you are unhappy, anxious or stressed. A cell's awareness is expressed in chemical reactions instead of words. No matter. The message comes through loud and clear."
Deepak Chopra, MD

With just a pound of weight loss, your blood sugar will begin to drop. If you need to lose weight, stop procrastinating and do it now to help prevent, reverse, or control your diabetes. For many of my clients, the most difficult part of getting healthy is getting started. Make the decision today—it will be the best decision of your life.

"I am a Type-2 diabetic, and they took me off medication simply because I ate right and exercised. Diabetes is not like a cancer, where you go in for chemo and radiation. You can change a lot through a basic changing of habits."
Sherri Shepherd

For more resources go to:
www.tracyherbert.com/book-resources

Chapter Notes / Action Items

Value of a Coach

"When the world says, 'Give up,' Hope whispers,
'Try one more time.'"
Unknown

Professional athletes, CEO's, Sales Executives, and people who want a better life have coaches.

Here are things to look for in a good coach:

- o Practice what they preach.
- o Has good communication skills.
- o Provides applicable information.
- o Not a friend, but someone who can help you reach your health goals.
- o An accountability partner.
- o Understands the value of team effort and allows client to explore ways to be successful.
- o Provides valuable and accurate information.
- o Understands what client is trying to accomplish.
- o Is excited and passionate for your personal growth.
- o Will help client focus on today and the future.
- o Asks for and expects a commitment.
- o Is an active listener.
- o Can empathize with client.
- o Make sure the fit is right with regards to personality.
- o Puts you at ease.
- o Seeks information by asking pertinent questions.
- o Allows the client to do the work by setting goals.

o Find a coach who is passionate and knowledgeable about the health goals you are trying to reach.

Remember you are not in this alone! Take a deep breath and remember it's not too late.

"Everybody dies, but not everybody lives."
A Sachs

Don't lose hope!

If your goal is to prevent, reverse, or control your diabetes check out my website for additional information.

www.tracyherbert.com

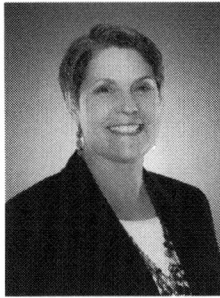

Goals to Accomplish

Actions Items	Date to Accomplish

40225815R00066

Made in the USA
San Bernardino, CA
14 October 2016